Who's Co

Responding to Elderly People who are Confused

by

Marilyn Harvey

ISBN 0 948680 19 9

The Author

Marilyn Harvey, currently an Independent Consultant in Social Care, started her career as a nurse at the West Suffolk Hospital. In 1984 she qualified as a Social Worker and practised in Essex as a specialist worker in mental health. The Author's interest in the subject of this book stems primarily from her experience as a practitioner in a psychiatric hospital, and more recently from her work as a trainer and In-House Development Worker for "Elders First", with Home Carers and Residential Practitioners.

© Marilyn Harvey 1990

Acknowledgements

I wish to thank:

- Participants who attended the "Who's Confused?" workshops initiated by "Elders First", Suffolk Social Services Department. They have strongly influenced the way this book has been written.

- Maureen Saunders, for editing this book, and for always demonstrating great patience and support during the writing process.

- Caroline Tisdall, Co-ordinator of "Elders First", whose skill and experience in enabling people to further realise their potential has made this book possible.

- Mary Macer and Lindsey Bickers, for their typing and secretarial support in seeing this book through its various draft stages.

Marilyn Harvey *October 1990*

Contents Guide

Preface		5
Chapter 1	What is Confusion?	7
Chapter 2	Understanding Challenging Behaviours	16
Chapter 3	The Carers' Perspective	25
Chapter 4	Reality Orientation	35
Chapter 5	Developments in Service Provision	43
Chapter 6	Your Questions Answered	51
Bibliography		58

Appendices

1	Useful Organisations	59
2	Useful Books about Practical Aspects of Care	61
3	Useful Publications about Finance	62

Index 63

Preface

"Who's Confused?" has been compiled for carers and workers who assist elderly people with their day-to-day living. This book is not intended to be an instruction manual about how to manage elderly people; neither does it reflect a complete study about the subject of 'Confusion'. Its aim is to increase the reader's understanding while offering factual information and practical ideas about how to maximise self-respect and independence with those individuals who experience short and long term deterioration of mental capabilities.

This book emerged from a series of workshops co-ordinated by Elders First, Suffolk Social Services Department's training and development agency for staff who work with older people. These workshops brought together individuals whose experiences as workers with elderly people were diverse and complementary. The participants' contributions to the workshops and to my learning enabled me to produce this material in book form more quickly than would have been possible had I been working alone.

The opening chapter challenges people to consider confusion using a multi-dimensional framework and outlines of case studies. Readers are introduced to the variety of conditions that can cause acute and/or chronic confusional states.

The book continues by giving insight into the effects of confusion on the individual's behaviour. Attention is given to the significance of wandering, inappropriate incontinence, aggression, loss of inhibition, hallucinations and delusions.

Anecdotes from those involved in caring for and living with elderly confused people explore the reactions of the carers to the behaviours exhibited, and the impact of such on the elderly person.

Having developed the scenario, the book then draws on the basic tenets of reality orientation, memory aids and reinforcement theories with the aim of stimulating carers and workers to think about the part they can play in orientating people who are confused and, where possible, helping to maintain predictable routines.

Special attention is given to the concept of multi-disciplinary practice. Outlines of the roles of the Psychogeriatrician, the Community Psychiatric Nurse, the Local Authority Social Worker, General Practitioner, Home Carers and Voluntary Organisations are explored.

The book concludes by recording questions asked by Carers and attempts to provide helpful guidelines and answers, together with an outline of the law as it relates to people who are confused.

Chapter One

What is Confusion?

The term "confusion" is one that is frequently used today to describe symptoms ranging from mild memory loss to acute or chronic disorientation; it is one that most of us can relate to. Confusion describes a state of mind. For whatever reason, it is concerned with diminished thinking power: perhaps about the time of the day, the day of the week, the whereabouts of a misplaced object or when a friend or person of significance was last seen, etc. Such disorganised thinking is an experience that many readers can identify with. With hindsight we recognise the antecedent as being related to tiredness, stress, physical illness, or hearing some bad news, and so on. Our experiential perception about this term is that it is usually a transient phase that is an integral part of life's events.

When linked to elderly people, however, the term "confusion" often takes on a different meaning. Historically, a confused state has often been regarded as the manifestation of "senility" or "becoming demented". Despite the fact that our experiences tell us it is a symptom that could indicate a number of different conditions, there is still a tendency to presuppose that an elderly person who becomes confused is suffering from a deteriorating mental condition, i.e. dementia, and that little can be done to treat or cure the problem.

"It is to be expected at her age".

"He has done well to have kept alert for so long. You have to expect him to deteriorate a bit at his age. It is understandable you are shocked, it has come on so suddenly with your father".

Anecdotes like this often echo conversations about people who experience differing degrees of mental deterioration. For some elderly people, diminished mental functioning is a living reality. Sometimes little can be done to cure or arrest the problem; but for many others, confusion is a symptom of a condition that can often be quickly and successfully treated.

The aim of this chapter is to outline a variety of conditions that cause acute and/or chronic confusional states. For ease of reading and learning, I shall consider the physical, emotional and mental influences and follow with a consideration of dementia. Within the context of practice, an individual may be experiencing one or more of these conditions. The worker must therefore understand the importance of a multi-dimensional assessment.

Physical Influences

The relationship between our bodies, minds and emotions is a complex one. The causes of any sudden change in behaviour and mental functioning can be numerous. An acute confusional state, particularly in elderly people, can frequently indicate physical causes, and these should be ruled out before determining alternative diagnosis. Examples of such conditions could include:-

Acute physical illnesses

Chest, bladder, etc. infections are common in the elderly population, the only signs to an onlooker being muddled thinking, disorientation and restlessness.

Ethel Ward, aged 83, had lived alone since her husband died two years previously. She looked after herself with the help of Home Care assistance once a week. She enjoyed good physical health and was mentally alert.

Over a three-week period she presented with symptoms of being disorientated and muddled about mealtimes. She had obviously not eaten. The house was beginning to look untidy, the clocks had stopped, no post had been taken out of the letter box and several days milk was still on the doorstep. Mrs Ward, in a very frightened and bewildered state, kept talking about people moving into her house. She fluctuated from being very angry to being very tearful when the Home Carer kept trying to tackle her in an attempt to understand what was going on. The crisis came when Mrs Ward failed to let the Home Carer in.

The GP visited and subsequently she was admitted to a psychogeriatric unit, diagnosed with an acute confusional state. Routine X-rays and blood tests confirmed that she had a chest infection and she was given a course of antibiotics and was quickly restored to normal health.

Impairment of bodily functions

Deteriorating senses, problems with eating, lack of certain vitamins, constipation, underactive or overactive thyroid, metabolic changes, kidney disease, liver disease, diabetes, anaemia, intercranial disorders etc., often have very direct effects on mental functioning. Sudden mental changes and changes over a period of weeks, and sometimes months, can indicate that the cause lies in physical disease.

Medication side-effects

Even the proper use of prescribed drugs to alleviate pain or to control some physical disorders can have very pronounced and unexpected side-effects. It need not necessarily be a newly-prescribed drug, but a cumulative effect of an existing drug that has been used over a period of time. Night sedation, for example, can leave some individuals confused and slow in their thinking during the day.

Alcohol Intoxication

Mr Compton, aged 69, was diagnosed as having early dementia. His thinking and memory were frequently muddled. Over a period of time he was less able to carry out daily tasks. People talked about him becoming a changed character - more withdrawn and less tolerant. He left his own home and moved to sheltered housing. One night his cooker caught fire and he was taken to hospital having been overcome by smoke fumes. There it was quickly discovered that he had been drinking heavily. Further investigations revealed that he had been drinking steadily for three years since his wife had died. With the appropriate support and help he reduced his drinking considerably, his memory improved and he was more able to care for himself. Persistent drinking and the consequent mental deterioration can mimic dementia in the similarity of symptoms presented.

Physical Trauma

A fall, a knock on the head, etc., should be carefully considered as an integral part of an assessment in acute confusional states.

All the foregoing conditions require full medical assessment and investigations to confirm the real cause of the mental deterioration. Given appropriate treatment and time, the person can often be restored to normal health. Delay in investigations and treatment can result in rapid deterioration which may necessitate some form of substitute care. It is important to remember that our response to the confused person can further exacerbate their problem. Where possible, individuals with acute confusional states should be enabled to remain in an environment that is familiar to them, thus reducing the likelihood of secondary confusion or disorientation as a result of a move.

Emotional Influences

Emotional traumas are not the most easily talked-about subjects in our culture. Even less exposed is the subject of grief. Many workers often feel unsure about the real nature of grief and what forms such a traumatic experience take. The combination of silence from the grieving individual and the worker who feels ill-at-ease about exposing the subject often results in the experience not being recognised as significant to behaviours that result from it.

Bereavement through the death of another significant person is a common experience for elderly people. Disorganised thinking, acute confusion, searching, wandering and outbursts of anger are all symptoms of a normal grief reaction. For some people, they may present for a short period soon after the death; for others, the symptoms may be more prolonged. As is often the case with bereaved individuals, they experience phases of acute grief followed by phases of appearing to be their ordinary selves. Muddled thoughts, chaotic feelings, unpredictable behaviours and emotional outbursts can come and go over a protracted period of time. The anniversary of a death, the deceased person's birthday, and Christmas are all times when mourning people can feel most vulnerable and often present with earlier grief symptoms. An elderly person who appears to be coping well may, for no apparent reason to the worker, suddenly develop signs of acute confusion, disorientation, restlessness, searching and wandering, etc.

The death of a beloved one is regarded as the most traumatic loss for most people. As we grow older, our grief is not only about the loss of another. We are faced more and more with our own ageing process and mortality. Getting older in itself is a grieving experience. Other losses frequently evoke strong grief reactions: for example, a change in surroundings, leaving one's own home to go into care, not being able to maintain independence and having a Home Carer to assist, diminished physical strength, and so on.

These experiences within themselves can sometimes be the root cause of an acute confusional state. Workers may have little time to explain in great detail what is happening or to listen patiently while a person talks through their changed world in order to make sense of it. Symptoms are all too often frequently unrecognised for what they really are and, sadly, the elderly person is seen "slipping" into a demented state and consequently becomes "a management problem".

Mental Influences

Anxiety

Anxiety and the feelings associated with it are ones that most readers can recognise; it is an emotional state common to all ages. Extreme forms of anxiety can affect normal physical and mental functioning.

Anxiety states in elderly people are not uncommon, although they are often overlooked as being the primary cause of impaired concentration, memory loss, sleep disturbance, disorientation, changed eating habits, etc. With appropriate treatment, an individual's ability to think clearly and accurately can be restored in a relatively short space of time. A person presenting with these symptoms may have a history of anxiety, although this is by no means always the case.

Depression

Depression is a diagnosis that is generally given to mood disorders. There are two well-documented kinds. The first, "reactive depression", is extremely common amongst elderly people. Symptoms can include intense feelings of sadness, worthlessness, low self-esteem, agitation, difficulty in going to sleep, poor appetite and sometimes weight loss. The cause is usually explainable, i.e. the individual is reacting to circumstances within their environment.

Grief reactions and reactive depression can appear very similar. Those who are isolated and unable to be supported in their grief are more vulnerable to this form of depression. Time spent simply talking to a supportive listener can help to lift the mood. Sometimes counselling may be necessary. Drug treatment may be required for a short period of time, but care should be taken to review regularly drug therapy for reactive depression. All too frequently elderly people are taking drugs long after there is any real need for them.

Age and attitudes about the inevitability of elderly people slowing down often distract workers from making thorough and proper assessments and thus failing to provide the helping resources at the appropriate time. The second type of depression is generally known as "endogenous". There appears to be no external cause for a sudden deterioration in mood, although circumstantial factors can precipitate the onset. It can be so severe that sufferers become unable to identify their mood.

Clinical signs and symptoms can be recognised: poor mental functioning and a low mood are often more pronounced in the morning; sleep disturbance is characterised by persistent early-morning wakening. Delusional thoughts, auditory hallucinations, weight loss, self-neglect, retardation of physical activity and mental functioning are also typical symptoms of this condition. There may well be a history of depressive illness, although this must not be taken for granted.

Psychiatric assessment needs to be sought promptly for an elderly person who presents with such symptoms. Both novices and experienced workers have sometimes mistaken depressive illness with dementia. It is essential to avoid this mistake. Neglecting to identify the depression, and thus not treating it, reinforces the problem for the sufferer, and the risk of attempted suicide is real.

Mrs Sanders, aged 70, had led a very active life. She retired at 65 from her job as a manager in the City and moved to a village. For no apparent reason she became preoccupied with the belief that she was physically ill and she could no longer do things as quickly as she used to. Thorough physical examination ruled out any physical cause. A few months later, she complained of not thinking clearly; she could not remember everyday things. She had given up many of her activities because the effort was too great. Her appetite was poor and sleeping became a problem inasmuch as she would have a few hours sleep and then wake up. Her GP put it down to old age and explained her sleep problems and lack of appetite as being associated with her not using up enough energy.

She became more distressed because she was unable to maintain her home properly and a home help was arranged. Eventually she cut her wrists. On admission to Casualty she was assessed as attention-seeking. Her relatives were advised that she was probably lonely and was showing early signs of dementia. She was persuaded to move into sheltered housing.

The theme that echoed this elderly lady was: "Why can't I do things?" No amount of effort enabled her to feel she had succeeded. Her physical movements became slower and she became more disorientated and withdrawn from everyday events. Once again she was told nothing could be done and, following this, she jumped out of a window, falling 16 feet. She suffered a cracked rib and was admitted to a psychogeriatric assessment ward.

A careful assessment and period of observation confirmed that she had been suffering from severe depression for a long period of time. Following successful treatment, she returned home. Her memory was fully restored and she became physically active again and resumed a normal independent life.

Paraphrenia

This is a form of mental illness that often starts in old age. The condition is mainly characterised by thought disorder. Early indicators may show themselves through suspicious and/or delusional thoughts mainly about other people in the immediate environment.

- Molly Mace, aged 76 years, suddenly started to bang on her neighbour's door late at night, accusing them of taking all her food.

- Dorothy regularly wrote to the police asking them to arrest the children on her estate whom she believed were plotting to break into her house. Her suspicion was based on the fact that a group of youngsters often stood opposite her house talking.

Some people experience hallucinations, i.e. they hear voices telling them to do things or commenting on what they are doing.

- Mrs Singh constantly heard voices in her head telling her the world was coming to an end. She had notes all over her house and on her front door asking God to protect her.

Some people who present with these kind of symptoms may have a history of mental illness.

The cause of paraphrenia is directly related to thought disturbance rather than to the intellect. Confusion and/or memory loss are not features of this illness *per se*. However, signs of deteriorating mental capabilities, such as confusion, may well be apparent due to the secondary problems caused by this condition. Sleep disturbance, particularly for those who are preoccupied with suspicious thoughts or voices in the night, can create changes in an individual's daily routine. This may present as disorientation in time. Tiredness and the distress that can mark the onset of this condition may be reflected in memory impairment and muddled thinking.

With specialist psychiatric help, assessment and accurate diagnosis, the individual can be treated successfully. In many cases people remain at home with ongoing drug therapy and the support of psychiatric services.

Dementia

There are two main kinds of dementia that affect elderly people.

1. Alzheimer's Disease

This is the most common form. Research shows that the disease destroys cerebral nerve cells, particularly those associated with memory. Unlike the other conditions outlined, the disease is neither treatable nor reversible. Deterioration of mental functioning is usually gradual. In the early stages it may be characterised by forgetfulness, mild confusion, agitation and loss of concentration. The striking feature of this disease is that the individuals will often have a very sharp recall of events that happened much earlier in his or her life but lack any memory retention about recent events. Aggression, wandering, disinhibition, incontinence, accusing people of taking things and nocturnal activity are amongst the many different kinds of behaviours that can manifest themselves as this disease develops.

As the disease progresses, marked personality changes accompany the increasing disorientation. Living with such disturbing changes brings enormous distress to both carer and the cared for.

2. Multi-Infarct Dementia

In this type of dementia, mental function is affected because oxygenated blood supplies to the brain are insufficient; therefore brain tissues die. The most likely medical explanation is hardening of the arteries. Individuals who have a history of arterial disorders, strokes or heart conditions are obviously more vulnerable to this form of dementia.

Unlike Alzheimer's disease, the onset can be sudden and individuals can present with acute confusion, florid symptoms of memory loss and disorientation. Many appear to experience some recovery in their mental functioning until the next episode. People suffering with this kind of dementia often fluctuate in their mental functioning and personality changes are often less pronounced. There is still no known way of reversing the brain damage that has occurred, although some measures can be taken to reduce the problems associated with the blood supply to the brain, thus slowing down the progress of the disease.

Dementia is one of the most devastating diseases of old age. Enabling sufferers to maintain as high a quality of life as is possible must remain the foremost goal for all those involved.

As stated at the beginning of this chapter, the term "confusion" often takes on a meaning of its own when linked to elderly people. In reviewing these outlines, you will recognise that a confused state is an indicator of a diverse range of conditions, the majority of which can be successfully treated. The challenge for all involved with elderly people is to suspend historical assumptions about what confusion has meant in favour of approaching the problem in a sequential way and thus, through careful assessment, provide appropriate services.

Chapter Two

Understanding Challenging Behaviours

As you read through these next few pages, you will notice that themes emerge as to why elderly confused people behave as they do. For some, particularly those who have lost the ability to communicate, their behaviour may be reflecting a basic need that is not being met. For others, particularly those with dementia, it often indicates that the person is no longer retaining knowledge about the social codes of conduct that govern conforming behaviour. They are unaware of what they are doing. However, unpalatable though it may sound, some elderly people can just be "being difficult". This may be particularly true of those who have a long history of personality problems. Equally, a behaviour could be a reaction to the way the individual is being treated by others.

Challenging behaviours can take a variety of forms. The aim of this chapter is to outline some of those behaviours that manifest themselves in elderly confused people whilst commenting on ways to approach the problems.

Wandering

Wandering is a common behaviour amongst people who are confused. You may encounter individuals who wander about their house all day with what appears to be no sense of purpose. Others may cause alarm to neighbours, families and the local community, looking "vulnerable" as they wander around their locality. A minority of individuals evoke overt panic in others. They wander into the road when a car is coming, or they are found walking about after dark and/or inappropriately dressed.

Wandering can generate a great deal of anxiety amongst carers and workers. In the past many institutions coped with this behaviour by using restraining chairs, drugs to sedate and/or admitting people to "secure" (locked) units. Some of these practices still pertain, although fortunately they are decreasing.

At first sight the activity of "wanderers" may look aimless. This is not usually the case. Seeking to understand the significance of a behaviour is an essential part in the process of determining the most appropriate way of responding to it. Wandering may be a signal about:-

Physical Needs

Elderly people with deteriorating mental capabilities often enjoy relatively good physical health. They need to burn up physical energy.

Mrs Russell lived in residential care. She experienced memory loss and on occasions appeared muddled around the home. She frequently wandered off after tea, her perception being that she was going for a walk. Staff perceived her behaviour as wandering and so they quickly caught up with her and brought her back. There was usually a scene with the resident becoming angry, resentful and restless for the rest of the evening. She was quickly labelled "difficult to manage".

The way we respond to one behaviour plays a significant part in subsequent behaviours. Vigilance and prompt action alleviated the carers' anxiety. They returned her to a safe place. However, this did not meet Mrs Russell's need to walk, and thus she became more difficult to manage. More often than not we react out of anxiety to protect and thus limit the quality of life. Mrs Russell was eventually taken out for a short walk each day and her wandering stopped. Her relationship with staff became a positive one rather than one of conflict.

Emotional Needs

As outlined in Chapter One, searching can be an important part of the bereavement process. Returning to places of significance is a way of getting closer to the person or a memory about something important that has been lost. The sad and/or happy feelings it evokes can have an important therapeutic purpose in helping a person make sense of their loss and re-adjust to a new way of life. "Wandering" is frequently concerned with working out feelings and this grief work should be encouraged. This form of wandering may perplex staff, particularly if they have insufficient knowledge of the individual's own life history. A confused person may not be cognisant as to the purpose of their behaviour and are, therefore, unable to communicate what they are doing.

If the underlying cause of the behaviour is predominantly concerned with grief, it can be particularly pronounced during the first year following a bereavement. Encouraging a person to work through these feelings will often prevent major long term behavioural problems. This form of wandering usually ceases once the grief work is accomplished.

Individuals who are diagnosed as suffering from dementia sometimes regress back into habits that were an integral part of their younger lives. As the short term memory diminishes, the longer term memories are sometimes brought into sharp focus. This might be manifest through behaviour. The individual sometimes acts out old habits, such as wandering off at 8 o'clock in the morning as if he is still going to work.

This kind of habitual wandering often proves problematic to resolve. Explanations may have little effect on a person with short term memory loss since, by the next day, they will have forgotten what you said and the life-long habit is likely to prevail.

Diverting the individual to a different activity can work with some people. Generally, the diversion has to be constant, often carried through over a long period of time before the wandering ceases. It is important to divert the individual at the time the old habit is acted out.

Wandering may appear inexplicable. For many people there is a purpose, even if it cannot be expressed or we cannot understand it.

Restraining, however sensitively done, is very traumatising for the individual concerned. It evokes intense inner conflicts, particularly if the individual is trying to act out ordinary needs, e.g. to exercise or grieve. Restraint will invariably force whatever need is being signalled to exhibit itself in more distorted ways, and thus behaviour becomes more difficult to manage. Alternatively it can turn inwards, resulting in withdrawal and depression.

Risk-taking behaviours such as wandering, fears that people will leave their cookers on, etc., are problematic to carers. The correct response is difficult to determine. Holding the tension between allowing an individual to expose themselves to untenable risk as opposed to ever-protective practices is a skilful task. Current policies and practices tend to reflect a shift in emphasis from being over-protective to allowing individuals to experience a degree of risk in order to maximise their quality of life.

Experience has taught me that there is still a tendency to speculate about the risks people are exposed to rather than testing out the reality. The latter might include, for example, "shadowing" a wanderer or, alternatively, letting them take the carer for a walk, giving an opportunity to observe what is done when they get to a kerb and whether they do know how to get home. All too often our anxieties prevent us from looking at levels of real risk in a systematic way; thus our judgments become clouded by speculative anxiety.

Inappropriate Incontinence

This is a term used to describe incontinence that generally has no physical cause. It is essential to eliminate physical causes for incontinence before considering other reasons.

Simple explanations can often be found for a person who may be incontinent without physical cause. A changed environment, for example, may mean the toilet is much further away from where the person sits than it was in their own home. Anxiety and emotional trauma may cause temporary incontinence. This often resolves itself with time, particularly if there is no history of incontinence.

Although not common, anger can be the root cause of such behaviour. This is not generally characteristic of incontinence related to a person who experiences acute and/or chronic confusion *per se*.

Those with dementia who are aware of their need to go to the toilet can become particularly distressed. On the way they forget what they intended to do and they either urinate or defecate in an inappropriate place. Such behaviours can burden the individual with a great deal of guilt and embarrassment. Afterwards they often realise what they have done. Allowing the person to share their feelings of guilt and embarrassment can help them to feel less isolated in their distress. Reassurance and understanding rather than impatience or disapproval help alleviate the deep feelings that people can experience.

For some individuals, incontinence may be a long term problem. Once a person's short term memory loss becomes very pronounced it may be impossible for them to retain details about where the toilet is. Memory reinforcers detailed in Chapter Four may help with this problem. For those in the later stages of dementia, incontinence problems may not be preventable. Managing the problem, by using incontinence aids, may be less distressing for the individual. Such a strategy should always be a last resort.

Incontinence can bring rewards, particularly for those individuals receiving a minimum amount of attention but needing or wanting more. Being helped to change into dry clothes, etc., secures private time and physical contact with the carers. Such needs are common to us all. This kind of attention-seeking is not usually a conscious act. However, such behaviours often evoke anger in carers who are already overworked. If this is the cause, it is often less time-consuming to give more attention to the individual for positive behaviour, and thus eliminate the work that goes with incontinence.

Incontinence is a complex subject in relation to elderly people. The causes can be partly physical, psychological, cognitive or simply a practical problem about no longer being able to undo their clothing. It is important to assess carefully and address the causes that can be treated before resorting to strategies that reduce the possibility of people maintaining independence over their toileting habits.

Aggression

This may take the form of verbal abuse or physical violence towards another person. Such behaviour is often particularly difficult for others. If the behaviour is seen as posing a personal threat, fear within can cloud the ability to assert the skills that are necessary to deal with the situation.

There are numerous reasons why people become aggressive. With elderly, confused people, causes can include:-

1. The fear of getting old, becoming dependent, not being able to understand what is going on around one, enforced changes through deteriorating health, not being understood; all these can be a tremendous threat to a person's autonomy. Such threatening situations often evoke more primitive behaviours.

2. The way a person has coped with stress in the past. "Learnt

aggression" is the term used to describe those who assert such behaviours as a way of coping with stress and/or life's problems that are not acceptable to them.

3. The way the individual is treated by others. The way we respond to people, coupled with their own personal problems, often exacerbates frustration and a sense of helplessness. Consequently the person "acts out".

Experience has taught me two important aspects about dealing with an aggressive outburst. The first is concerned with what the carer does when faced with the aggression. The second relates to considerations about long term management problems.

An important first step if confronted with aggression is to use skills likely to calm the individual and create a safe boundary.

a) Space and height - it is not advisable to get too close or tower over the aggressor. It can feel very intimidating and such actions are more likely to provoke further aggression.

b) Initial communication - ensure this is calm and empathetic. Let the person know that you have understood his/her anger, as this demonstrates your understanding and can help defuse the situation.

c) Appropriate response - elderly confused people are often frightened when showing aggression.

They will more often than not calm down if met with a calm, firm and understanding response rather than an impatient or angry reaction.

Longer term management strategies will need to be considered carefully, especially where there is a threat to other equally vulnerable elderly people. If the behaviour cannot be safely or sensitively managed in the existing environment, then it may be necessary and kinder to seek a more appropriate home for the aggressive individual.

Loss of Inhibitions

We are all familiar with the sight of an elderly, confused person appearing half-dressed, naked or starting to undress in public. These are embarrassing problems with which carers are frequently confronted.

Despite the concern they generate, particularly for those in the community, behaviours of this kind are rarely intended as a form of sexual exposure.

John Stewart, aged 75, had been dementing for four years and his ability to communicate had progressively diminished. He frequently took his trousers off in the residents' sitting room. "Why now?" was the question to which staff struggled to find an answer. After careful recording of the frequency of his behaviour and subsequent physical examinations, the staff learnt that he suffered with constipation. Physical pain, badly fitting clothing, forgetting where the toilet or bedroom is, may give rise to such behaviours. Careful consideration needs to be given to reactions to such behaviours.

If a person is trying to signal a need and, as a consequence of their behaviour, the need is met, the behaviour is likely to reoccur. Mr Stewart's reward for taking his trousers off in public was to be relieved of his constipation. We may not see it in those terms, but that is how he most likely experienced it.

Having identified a cause or causes for such inappropriate behaviour, it is essential to anticipate the need and, where possible, meet it before the behaviour occurs. An appropriate strategy with Mr Stewart would be to explore ways of preventing his constipation and pain.

As with all of the behaviours I indicated, there may be no logical explanation. Confrontation rarely works, particularly with those with dementia. Removing the person from the scene calmly may be the only way to manage the problem, as and when it occurs. Chapter Four will detail some memory aids to help individuals retain dress sense. These are particularly helpful if the cause of exposure relates to forgetting to put appropriate clothing on.

A minority of individuals may be expressing sexual frustration. If carers assess that the person does have awareness of what they are doing, then the use of some kind of boundary strategy may well alleviate the problem. For example, placing a person away from others when they exhibit the behaviour may solve the problem. Some Home Carers complain of clients who masturbate while they are there. Responses to such sensitive issues should, where possible, be determined by organisational guidelines rather than by any one individual.

Hallucinations and Delusions

As outlined in Chapter One, hallucination is the clinical term used to describe hearing imaginary voices or, in rare cases, seeing imaginary things or people. Delusions are concerned with a belief that is real to the individual but has no reality base outside that person's mind.

Symptoms such as these often leave carers feeling helpless about how to respond. There is a temptation either to collude with the bizarre thought patterns or to argue against them in an effort to convince the individual that their experience is not real.

There is little point in trying to convince a person who is experiencing bizarre thoughts or beliefs that they are not real. For the sufferer, they are a living reality and often extremely distressing.

The most appropriate way to respond to these symptoms is firstly to acknowledge that the experience may be real to them. This communicates understanding. Secondly, this should be followed up by stating that you cannot see or hear what they can. Remaining neutral is less likely to exacerbate the problem. Experience has taught me to exercise extreme caution with those who exhibit extreme paranoid reactions, e.g. "You are poisoning me". These individuals are often extremely frightened and inappropriate reactions can evoke aggression. As stated in Chapter One, it is important to seek medical help for these kinds of symptoms. They can be successfully treated with drug therapy and, where necessary, psychiatric help.

* * * * *

The behaviours outlined in this chapter are by no means exhaustive. They do attempt to underline the importance of exploring behaviours in a systematic way.

In the first place, it is essential to have information about the individual in the context of their own life history. For example, understanding their personality, coping styles and losses, etc., prior to the onset of their confusion helps to form an important picture in understanding their present behaviour.

Secondly, it is important to reflect on the stimuli that precipitate the behaviour. Looking at the way we behave towards an elderly confused person can often explain why they behave as they do. Particular attention should be paid to this in hospitals and residential homes. Residents can be exposed to a number of carers in any one day. This in itself presents problems for elderly confused people and they often react in different ways for different carers.

Thirdly, it is of great significance to explore the behaviour itself. More often than not, it is signalling a basic need. Anticipating the need and responding appropriately to it often results in the problem behaviour not manifesting itself.

Finally, we must look at the way the behaviour is responded to. The response will frequently be the force that nurtures the behaviour to repeat or eliminate itself. Consistent approaches and responses to behaviour need to be carefully thought out. It is essential that all carers reinforce the same response. This aspect of behavioural management is often the most problematic for carers with elderly confused people. Attitudes and values about how they should be treated are diverse. It is not uncommon to see a carefully devised behavioural plan sabotaged because some of the carers may not agree. They quietly get on and respond in ways that are most comfortable to them, rather than standing where the confused person stands. This can be unnecessarily distressing for the person who is confused.

Behavioural management with elderly confused people has proved to be a successful way of reducing a number of challenging behaviours. This is particularly true of those that reflect a need for physical, emotional and/or social attention.

Despite beliefs to the contrary, many people with dementia still have a capacity to learn and respond to behavioural programmes of care. Efforts made by carers to test out different strategies over a period of time have often improved the quality of life for the sufferer and decreased the carer's workload. It has to be acknowledged that a minority of people who are severely demented may not respond. Nonetheless, it is important to try, rather than to presuppose the person is no longer capable.

Chapter Three

The Carers' Perspective

So far the primary focus of this book has been the individual and those conditions that may cause a confused phase or permanent mental deterioration and the behaviours that may result from it. Most readers would readily accept that such conditions, however transient or permanent, can be traumatic to the individual. In the early stages people can often be bewildered by their own unpredictable behaviour, irritated with themselves for not being able to do the things the way they used to, embarrassed and frightened about the future.

Less well recognised and even less well documented are the experiences of those who are in different ways interconnected to the individual who is confused, i.e. husband, wife, partner, children, other family members, a close friend or a caring neighbour.

This chapter attempts to bring into sharper focus experiences that are felt by those who are close to somebody who has been diagnosed with dementia.

Responses and adjustments to dementia are many. To my knowledge, there appear to be no sequential patterns of reactions to draw upon which might provide a framework for workers to understand the experiences for families, relatives and/or friends. Reactions to such conditions are numerous and often depend upon variables associated with personality traits, the quality of the attachment to the individual concerned, patterns of interaction, social circumstances, the support that is available, the way that the disease manifests itself and perceptions about the strengths and limitations of the labelling process. Each person's experience is unique to them in the context of their relationship to the individual with dementia.

The following anecdotes from relatives and friends by no means illuminate the full range of experiences that people feel. They attempt to alert the reader to the reactions that dementia can evoke in others whose familiar patterns of living may also be altered by the disease.

A Neighbour's View

"We used to get on so well as neighbours. We met 60 years ago when we both moved into the terrace. A few months ago she started to go a bit funny, not talking to me. She couldn't find her way to the shop. I was so upset about that. I asked her what I had done, she couldn't remember that she hadn't talked to me. One night she kept banging on the walls and shouting. I was so scared that I got my son out. He went after her and was cross, she wouldn't stop doing it. I expect he was only trying to protect me. After that I found it hard to be in the house alone. I wasn't sure what she was going to do next. The doctor gave me some sleeping tablets but I was still frightened during the night. Yet when she passed my house, during the day, I kept wanting to say hello to her and invite her in like we used to do. Every day we would just pop in on each other. It was nice because it passed the time a bit. I just couldn't bring myself to go in any more. I didn't know what to say when she said funny things. Sometimes she'd cry; I felt awful; then all the wall-banging, I was frightened she might hit me if I went back. It's strange, us not popping in on each other. If only I hadn't called my son, perhaps I should have just ignored it."

The questions that went through this neighbour's mind and the mixture of feelings that she experienced are ones often expressed. Fears about the unpredictable nature of her neighbour's behaviour forced her to avoid a situation that she felt helpless about. Her way of dealing with the situation also stirred within her feelings of sadness about changing a longstanding routine with a friend, of guilt about not knowing how to help and sometimes of regret about calling her son: "if only I hadn't done that..."; "If only I hadn't called my son...."

"If only ..." is one way in which people try to make sense of their own reactions towards elderly people who are behaving in unpredictable ways.

"If only somebody would tell us how we can help her, then we'd know what to do."

"If only the police could keep an eye on him at night; it's such a worry having somebody like that next door."

"If only he would just agree to go into a home; he would be safer there."

The proposed Community Care Act that is intended to underpin social care sharply reflects an integrationalist philosophy. The focus is on further developing community care resources to enable the majority of individuals who need social and health care support to remain in their own living environments. Such a shift in emphasis, away from residential and hospital care, poses some interesting questions about the role of the informal carers of those who have dementia.

Traditionally, service provision has tended to be targeted towards the individual who is seen to be 'the problem'. More recently, efforts have been made to hold the tension between, on the one hand, individuals and their rights and, on the other, the needs of neighbours, families and friends. Phased or short term residential care, to offer regular periods of relief for carers, support groups, day care facilities and a more flexible Home Help Service are becoming a more established part of the service provision within many geographical areas throughout the country. These developments have enabled many of those who were previously cared for away from the public eye to remain in the community.

Sadly, in my experience, similar developments in education with regard to increasing the carers' understanding and knowledge about those individuals previously segregated, are not yet so widely established. For some people, participating in caring still remains an option they cannot consider. Perceptions and understanding are sometimes based on fear, lack of knowledge and a real lack of confidence about supporting vulnerable people, whether they be family, friend or neighbour.

Whatever the reasons motivating carers, their real worth, in terms of enabling vulnerable people to remain in the community, fully justifies service provision that can meet the carers' needs for knowledge, skills development and support. Regardless of legislation, there will always remain the uncomfortable dilemma of weighing up the needs and rights of the individual who is confused, alongside those of the people living in close proximity who may also live with the increased risk of harm or damage.

Emotional Reactions to Dementia

"I hadn't really registered what the doctor meant when he told me my husband had got dementia. He didn't seem too bad to me. Sometimes

he got muddled and it became more noticeable when he found it hard to remember things. I expected that at our age. But one day it all hit home. He came indoors and kept asking where his wife had gone. I felt sick. It was as if the person I had married had died, yet the mechanics of eating, sleeping and living together continued as if nothing had happened. You cannot explain it to people easily. The next day he knew I was his wife again. People would have thought I had gone funny if I told them that I had suddenly felt widowed. After all, there he was sitting in the chair at home as large as life. On his good days he remembered things so clearly. Then I would think that he was getting better. Other days he was like a total stranger to me. I used to feel sad, even despairing; I could no longer leave him alone. Yet anger often coloured my sadness; I would get cross and shout at him. My husband has been sick for 18 months now. I feel less dazed by it all. I try to laugh when he doesn't recognise me. Sometimes I still hope he will recover. Other times I feel so depressed about the future. It does feel easier than it was, since I am getting used to his unpredictable behaviour and we now have a different routine."

It is difficult to generalise about the impact a diagnosis of dementia has on a close relative. Some relatives may have lived with the early signs of the disease long before a medical assessment and determinate diagnosis has been made. Some adjustments may have already been made to compensate for failing short term memory, unfinished sentences and repetitive speech. Some aspects of personal care, dress, etc., have been gradually taken over by the carer. Slowly comes the painful awareness that the condition is irreversible. For some close relatives a diagnosis brings an initial sense of relief.

"I was petrified the doctor was going to tell me he had a brain tumour."

"Anything is better than being told she had gone mad."

Parallel to this sense of relief can come also feelings of numbness and sometimes shock, as the carer is faced with the realisation that dementia is incurable.

It is also not unusual for close relatives to enter into phases of denial concerning the irreversibility of the condition. Feelings of having to constantly care, together with the grief that the carer may feel, can be overwhelming. Phases of denial can be helpful, particularly during the early stages, as the close relative gradually learns to adapt to the reality of a chronic and deteriorating disease. As they gradually come to terms with the changes and with the prognosis, phases of denial become less and coming to terms with the reality of the situation becomes more obvious.

The last case study demonstrates how the relative's feelings can fluctuate. These feelings are further reinforced by one characteristic of the disease: it is also usually a fluctuating one.

"On the good days he remembered things so clearly. Then I would think he was getting better. Other days he would be like a total stranger, not knowing who I was...."

The impact of the disease is painfully reinforced when the individual affected does not recognise their loved ones or they do something so totally out of character. The losses for the carer can be pronounced and multiple. For some it can feel like the death of a person who is close. Yet the situation demands that a different alliance is created between them.

Literature on the subject of loss and change, such as that by Colin Murray Parkes (1972) and Elizabeth Kubler Ross, authenticates those reactions described above as being an integral part of a normal grief reaction. Such authors also bring into sharp focus a range of other different emotions that are a usual part of grieving.

Anger

Anger is a feeling that carers often talk about as being one of the most difficult feelings to deal with. There can be anger about:-

1. The *diagnosis* itself; "why us?" ... "Why can't the doctor do more?"
2. Some of the *behaviours* that characterise dementia; "Why does she keep going out half-dressed; it's embarrassing; the neighbours will think I don't care; I get so cross with her for doing such stupid things."
3. *Oneself* as a carer; "If only I didn't have a heart condition then I could do more for him...." Being angry and frustrated with oneself

is a particular problem for elderly partners as often they too may be experiencing physical health problems that prevent them caring at the level they may need or want to.

One of the biggest difficulties about sharing strong feelings of anger is concerned with how the person you are talking to might react.

"I was so very angry with my husband when he became doubly incontinent all the time. He was admitted to hospital. That's what separated us. It's hard being alone. I couldn't even tell my own daughter how angry I was with him. I thought she might have taken it the wrong way. I tried to explain it once to the District Nurse. All she could say was 'he couldn't help it and I should try not to think about it too much'. All I needed was for people just to let me talk about being really angry, for a few minutes, without their comments. I just felt so alone in my angry world every time the nurse said 'he can't help it'. At times I remember being frightened of my own angry feelings. I just wanted to talk to others to see if they felt like it too."

Guilt

Guilt is a common feeling for carers; intense guilt about feeling angry towards somebody who is defined as ill can be very real.

"I get really cross and shout at her when the shopkeeper tells me she has not paid for the goods. I feel awful to keep shouting at her, because I know she can't help it. What can I do?"

"Every night he wanders around the house. I get so tired and cross; it's exhaustion I think. He just cries when I shout. Sometimes he says "sorry". Other times he tries to hit out at me. The doctor says shouting at him wouldn't help. That leaves me feeling I have been really cruel."

Feelings of guilt often become very pronounced at the stage when a carer may need a rest themselves and have to accept short term or permanent alternative care for their partner, relative, friend or neighbour. Feeling a sense of failure about needing to use alternative accommodation for the person who is demented is not uncommon, however hard the carer may have tried to look after their relative at home.

"I never feel at ease when she is away. I hate leaving her in the home. She doesn't understand I will come back for her. She always cries and clings to me. When she returns home she's always more confused. I just couldn't keep her at home without the breaks every so often. The breaks give me a bit of a rest. All the time I keep thinking I shouldn't do it to her. I know she hates it."

There is often a temptation amongst workers to smooth over the real feelings that need to be expressed by the carers when they place their relatives in alternative accommodation.

"You mustn't worry, she's in good hands with us..."

"You shouldn't feel guilty about leaving him. That's what we are here for."

There is a fine line between offering reassurance to relatives and suppressing their real feelings. Listening, encouraging people to share their feelings, and reassuring them their reaction is usual is most likely to communicate empathy, reassuring the carer that their loved one is being left with those who have understanding and sensitivity.

Helplessness

These feelings often accompany the gradual realisation that a relative may need additional help. This may be in the form of short term care, and/or domiciliary visits from community support services to enable the individual affected to remain at home for as long as possible and preserve some semblance of family life.

Having underlined some of the feelings that manifest themselves in individuals who are faced with loss and or change, I want again to stress the fact that individual reactions will be variable. Sometimes close relatives will want time and space to reflect on their experiences and understand what is happening. Enabling the expression of strong emotions may be the most helpful way to support an individual in dealing with an unpredictable future. For others, openly expressing their feelings may not be the most appropriate way for them to deal with the transitions to which a disease such as dementia can expose them to. Parkes (1972) writes: "There is an optimal level of grieving which varies from one person to another. Some will cry and sob, others will betray their feelings in other ways. The important thing is for the feeling to emerge into consciousness. How they appear on the surface may be of secondary importance..."

Traditionally the focus for understanding reactions to loss and change has tended to reflect individualistic perspectives, e.g. the reaction of the grieving individual. More recently, there has been a growing interest in seeking to understand individuals in the context of a family group and the part that each person plays in ensuring that the family system functions as a whole unit. The implications of this approach, in terms of using it as a practice tool, are way beyond the scope of this book. Nonetheless drawing on some of the basic tenets of family work approaches can help workers more fully understand areas of vulnerability for those who are in a forced changed situation. In such an incidence, a family member might not be able to sustain his or her part in ensuring that the family system functions as it had prior to the onset of a disease.

The role that family members play in relation to each other is an important area of study for workers who try to understand families as a whole. This can be looked at from a number of different perspectives.

"Up until my husband became confused, he always made all the decisions for us. He had looked after all the money and our affairs since we were married. It was very difficult for me to take over. I just didn't know where to start. It threw us into chaos. I was so petrified about how we were going to survive financially; I was tired and worried about his health. My son took all the money worries off me in the end; it seemed the right thing to do at the time. I am not sure now I feel so dependent on him."

This is not an uncommon scenario of an elderly couple who are faced with the traumas of dealing with the unpredictable. This woman's husband played a vital role in their system, a role that in the circumstances they faced she felt unable to take over. In seeking a solution, other roles are reversed also. Her son, the person who has historically depended on his parents, becomes the dependable person in the system to ensure the family continues to function at an economic level.

Disequilibrium, in relation to role and function at an economic level, obviously creates additional stress. Where possible, carers should not be encouraged to make any permanent decisions about changes whilst they are trying to cope with the acute pressures that adjusting to the role of 'caring for' brings. Once the acute phase of adjustment is over, they may well have the capacity to learn new skills and take on 'roles' that will increase their autonomy.

Other functions and roles that commonly cause disequilibrium in families faced with forced change are concerned with decision-making, the ways in which problems are solved, boundaries and the environment.

Decision-making

Who is the decision-maker in the system? Is it a shared role or are decisions usually made by one member? It may prove problematic, initially, if the main decision-maker is the individual affected by the disease or the role has been a shared one. Confidence building for the carer, together with skills acquisition, will serve to help them to test out their untapped potential as a decision-maker. Some carers may prefer to hand this role on to other family members; others may respond to the appropriate encouragement and support in becoming decision-makers in their own right.

The ways that problems are solved

Attempting to understand previous patterns of problem-solving may well help the worker appreciate how a family might deal with an individual who has dementia. Faced with loss and change, the majority of people use their past coping styles to deal with current trauma, although some individuals concerned may use the opportunity to discover new ways of dealing with the new situations.

Boundaries

Attempting to understand the extent to which the members of families are dependent on or independent of each other emotionally will help workers to more fully understand the emotional transitions that carers may have to make. The autonomy of the carer may well be more difficult to realise if their emotional relationship to the person with dementia has been extreme and over-dependent.

Links with the environment

Which family member usually initiates this? This may be a particularly important area of concern with elderly people whose contact with others is limited through lack of mobility, etc., or because they have chosen to be a very insular couple.

Forced changes through chronic and deteriorating illness can be more fully understood if it is placed in both the context of:-

        a) the family system, and

        b) the individuals concerned.

Prioritising of approaches is sometimes a real temptation for workers, particularly if they have preferred ideologies about the way problems are explored and understood and also feel tenacious that one approach is more profitable than another. Both perspectives form important assessment indicators. They enable some clearer understanding about aspects of individual and family functioning that may be strengths to the people involved in a family difficulty. Equally they may help people to understand potential and actual areas of vulnerability.

Chapter Four

Reality Orientation

This chapter describes one way of assisting elderly confused people with their day-to-day living. It sets out to highlight the theory and practice of reality orientation, whilst illustrating some techniques that can be used:

    a) with individuals and/or groups,

    b) in people's own homes and/or in a group environment, e.g. residential homes or hospitals.

During the past ten to fifteen years, Reality Orientation techniques have excited growing interest amongst carers and workers. It has to be stressed, however, that it may take a long time for these techniques and the resources they demand to be budgeted for as an integral part of the basic provision for those in need. Prior to the techniques being practised in this country, they were researched and well used in the USA.

The techniques that will be described in this chapter are by no means the only 'enabling tools' to assist elderly people; equally the techniques are not exclusive to that group. For example they are often used with:-

■ Individuals who experience disorientation and memory loss following a serious head injury.

■ People who experience acute and/or chronic disorientation through sensory deprivation, i.e. disabilities associated with hearing, sight, touch and/or lack of stimulation through social isolation and/or social withdrawal.

The philosophical principle that underpins Reality Orientation is concerned with the empowering of individuals, who are confused or memory-impaired, to maximise their own normal functioning. This philosophy encourages methods of working which enable elderly persons to maintain their level of physical, emotional, social and cognitive functioning for as long as possible.

For those who have experienced disorientation and memory loss over a protracted period of time, Reality Orientation techniques have the potential for people to re-learn forgotten responses.

"She's beyond all that sort of thing now; she hasn't got a clue; she's been like it for weeks. The workers do their best; they keep her clean and comfortable".

"Poor old thing, she doesn't know her dress from her petticoat. She has to be dressed every day now; I am not having her going down the shop dressed funny; it's an embarrassment to this household. What's the point in starting to put her clothes in the right order for her so she can continue to dress herself? It wouldn't work. Anyway she's been the independent sort all her life; it will be nice for her if we take over now. She is 87 years."

Variations of this theme about not testing out whether practical solutions could work are often echoed about those who have been labelled with dementia. Understandably, the morbid elements that are apparent with this disease can colour carers' enthusiasm to test out techniques that may improve quality of life, on a day-to-day basis.

Reality Orientation is a way of working which aims to provide a series of regular and reinforcing stimuli that counteracts the problems caused by memory loss and/or confusion. The stimuli can take numerous forms, for example, information, pictures, images, activities and routines. It is important, however, to ensure that the stimuli chosen correlate to the actual impairment of the individual whose functioning is affected. This ensures that the individuality of each person is respected. A stimulus can be an interfering imposition if not sensitively used. For ease of reference I have listed the stimuli under two categories, namely environmental and interpersonal.

Environmental Stimuli

Differentiating areas of an individual's home and/or a residential establishment draws attention to their functional purpose and can provide a consistent and reinforcing aid to orientation. Imaginative use of lighting, pictures and/or clear labels on doors can offer guidance to those who may feel lost. For example, putting labels on drawers and cupboards indicating their contents assists in reminding people where things are kept; clear information on cookers, reminding an individual to turn it off, may reduce risk. The challenge for those who are involved with people who may be helped by Reality Orientation is to adapt environments imaginatively.

Another important way of enhancing a stimulating environment is to make full use of time-recording items, for example, ensuring that clocks have clear faces, that calendars can be easily seen, and that they are of the kind that record the day of the week, besides the date and the month. Aids of this kind can help people to keep track of time. It is also important to ensure the written word is large enough to compensate for those with failing sight.

Modifying environments in the ways described above may appear to be a fairly straightforward and practical way of maximising people's autonomy. In some ways it is so straightforward that it poses questions as to why the environments of more people who are confused are not more stimuli-sensitive. One answer of course may be that the individual in need does not want their environment adapted. Experience has taught me that these methods of work can also pose problems for workers and carers. The common themes echoed to me are:-

> "It's treating them like children."
>
> "It looks awful having all those labels about the place."
>
> "Turning the home into an infants' classroom may help the demented residents, but it's a huge insult to the residents that are not demented."

Paradoxically, 'time' is of the essence in this kind of situation. On the one hand, adapting an environment at the time appropriate to the person's failing memory offers the opportunity for them possibly to remain independent longer. On the other hand, attitudinal change for those who feel uneasy about the techniques also demands time and understanding. This is particularly true for some relatives. Parallel to their loved ones becoming affected by severe memory loss, they too are often trying to come to terms with the changes this may demand. Adapting a person's home may reinforce a sense of permanence about their condition. As described in Chapter Three, people often need time to absorb and come to terms with a diagnosis such as dementia.

My own response to this kind of paradox consists of:

1. acknowledging and attempting to communicate empathy for the person who feels uneasy about the techniques regardless of what the dis-ease is about or whether it is justified or not. The feeling is real for them.

2. encouraging them to explore what kind of environmental stimuli they use as memory aids. People usually echo similar objects e.g. clocks, watches, radio, TV, diaries, labels, etc.,

The purpose of this kind of dialogue is to bring into sharper focus the way that most people depend on a reinforcing environmental stimuli to help maintain and reinforce a sense of routine and, to a greater or lesser extent, predictability. In my experience, this kind of dialogue has helped relatives and carers to appreciate more fully the importance of accentuating those 'reminding and reinforcing tools' for those who are disorientated or memory-impaired.

Interpersonal Stimuli

Building on the environmental stimuli and reinforcing reality through interpersonal communication can be done in a number of different ways. The regularity and intensity of this kind of communication depends partly on the level of need that is presented and partly on the resources that are available.

Capitalising on Existing Interpersonal Contact

In this level of intervention, an important part is played by people such as home carers, residential workers and relatives who have regular contact with the individual experiencing problems in functioning.

In the early stages of dementia, for example, a person's memory, concentration and orientation abilities fluctuate from being, on the one hand, very alert and, on the other, very confused and forgetful. Therefore encouraging the person to make the most of using adapted environmental stimuli often helps to delay mental deterioration.

Constantly referring to them by name reinforces their identity; maximising existing social interaction by encouraging them to talk more provides a stimulus; ensuring when you leave that you tell them the date, day and time you are returning keeps people alert to time. Where possible, encourage the person to keep a diary and help them write in it; keep a record of callers. When they experience a phase of being disorganised in their thinking, it can be referred to by them or somebody else. Enabling them to write down the events and visitors themselves further reinforces orientation and encourages concentration. There is often a temptation to take over, even in small ways: "I'll do the shopping list". This is particularly the case when the carer's time feels very precious. With those who have deteriorating mental capabilities, and/or are in the early stages of dementia, situations can be created to enable people to use their skills in:-

- decision-making
- concentration
- memory-reinforcement

This will often help to, at least, maintain some level of functioning. Although forgotten responses can be revived in some people, it may be more helpful to keep the mind as exercised as possible during the early stages of the disease.

Intense Programmes of Reality Orientation

These tend to take the form of constantly orientating information. On every occasion a carer interacts with the individual who is confused, they remind and reinforce reality.

The purpose of each communication is to:-

1. Reinforce information that is helpful in sensitising the individual to current everyday facts, e.g. "There is a lot of cloud about for July; it's normally much sunnier at this time of year" - gives more information about the time than "Isn't it cloudy today?"

   Relatives and carers will obviously have their own styles of talking. The important theme is concerned with maximising each piece of information that is exchanged.

2. Encourage a response from the individual. This enables them to exercise their social and interactive skills in a reality-based context.

Intense reality orientation programmes of the kind described above demand that the orientating stimuli and responses are co-ordinated. The success or failure of this kind of intervention relies heavily on the consistency of interaction in relation to both the information that is given and the response that is offered to the person concerned.

The most usual practice is for the carer to positively acknowledge appropriate responses made by the individual who is confused, but ignoring any confused talk by diverting the conversation to something else that is closer to reality.

Reality Orientation programmes that are intense need to be accepted by all the carers involved. They should therefore be carried out as an integral part of every routine within the environment of those who are being stimulated. Therefore, where possible, the carers involved need to have an appreciation for:-

1. The importance of work that may do no more than maintain present levels of functioning. Where memory impairment can't be improved, the aim should be to prevent it deteriorating further.

2. The significance of small change.

Also, they must acquire an understanding of the importance of:-

1. Communicating information clearly and in an uncomplicated way.

2. Using short sentences.

3. The worth of constant repetition, where appropriate.

4. Touch as a powerful communicating tool.

5. A team approach.

6. Ensuring that the individual succeeds, however small the task.

Group Reality Orientation

Another way to offer interpersonal orientation and stimulation is through the use of groupwork activities. These techniques can be very useful in hospital settings and residential establishments.

The purpose of group Reality Orientation is similar to the other techniques outlined above. Stimulation, learning and re-learning forgotten responses is the primary aim of such activities. They allow people to participate and, more importantly, the method can be an enjoyable one for those involved.

More detailed information about group work and of the activities that can be used in groups can be found in the bibliography and appendices at the back of the book.

For example, name games may be played by a small group of six to eight people. The individual's own identity is constantly reinforced and so too are the names of those people they may be living with. Singing and music activities firstly offer stimulation and, secondly, opportunities to recall memories and songs from the past. Besides exercising memory and thinking skills, activities that stimulate thoughts and memories of the past have an important therapeutic value for those who have sharp recall of long term rather than short term memories.

Activities that evoke memories of past events and individual's own life histories can assist a person who is confused to make some sense of the present; they can use their long term memories to help reinforce their identity and who they are in relation to others who have played an important part in their lives. Working alongside somebody, helping them to do a life story book, for example, often helps to restore a person's self-esteem. They feel their memories about their life, who they were, where they lived and what they did, etc., are valuable enough for others to listen to. Exercises such as this also help carers to learn about the individual who is confused. An understanding of a person's life, as they perceive it, has important value, particularly if they should become so memory-impaired that their life becomes totally dependent on others.

Discussion groups about different topics that have meaning to the elderly generation, current affairs and/or other subjects of interest can exercise concentration, communication skills and also keep people alert to the wider world.

Whatever the group activity, preparation is important. Care should be taken in selecting the right people for the group. If an individual is unable to succeed in the activities, this can further reinforce a low self-esteem. Ensure that the necessary equipment is available, e.g. blackboard, overhead projector, pictures, etc. The value of the intent can be lost on people who are experiencing severe memory loss and confusion if the external stimuli fail to at least begin to compensate for the deteriorating mental capabilities of those involved.

* * * * *

As stated earlier in this chapter, the philosophical principle that underpins Reality Orientation is concerned with empowering individuals, who are confused and/or memory impaired, to maximise their normal functioning. I would like to emphasise the words 'their normal functioning'. Sometimes carers and workers have experimented with these techniques and have been disappointed and cynical about the results. The real problem may not be rooted in the methods used but in the assessment of the individual's normal functioning prior to the onset of their deteriorating mental capabilities. For example, if a person has always been a loner, this should be respected. A socialisation programme which aims to stimulate may be inappropriate to somebody's preferred living style and/or personality.

There is a real risk when working with people who are elderly and confused that carers impose standards of functioning that are totally alien to the vulnerable individual.

Chapter Five

Developments in Service Provision

Despite myths to the contrary, the majority of people with deteriorating mental capabilities live in the community. More often than not they are assisted or totally cared for by relatives and/or other informal support networks. Many of these people may never request a service from the official agencies; accurate statistics about the growing numbers of elderly people with deteriorating mental capabilities and/or dementia are difficult to determine. Some people do not request a service because they do not have a need to. Sadly, for many others, the problem is associated with a real lack of knowledge about what is available or how to access the help they may require. People have a tendency to carry on, or muddle on, for months and even years until a crisis emerges.

The problems associated with accessing resources can be very pronounced for ethnic minority groups whose knowledge about services may be limited. Non-English speaking people may be further disadvantaged in their search for knowledge about available services, particularly in those areas where the only form of written information is in English. A great deal of information about service provision presupposes that people can read English.

Often it is a crisis that is the precipitating factor forcing people into contacting the helping services. Service provision in this country tends to be 'reactive' rather than 'proactive'. For those with dementia, the later and more problematic stages of their illness are often reached before any help is given. Assessments about real functioning are coloured by the crisis. Care programmes to maximise opportunities for people to retain their autonomy are often thwarted because the expertise that is available is often not connected to the person in need, at the appropriate time. There are a number of obvious reasons for this.

1. Traditionally, a common response to those with dementia has been the use of some form of custodial care, i.e. admission to hospital or a residential home. Such strategies may have alleviated the social crisis, but practitioners are learning that this kind of approach has

often exacerbated the problem for some individuals with dementia. Symptoms of confusion, disorientation, etc., become more pronounced. The likelihood of rehabilitating a person back into the community becomes more problematic. The already limited accommodation that is available becomes inaccessible to others. Beds have often been filled on a long term basis with those who were admitted, during a crisis, for intended short stays, but they end up being unable to return home due to the secondary problems caused by changing the person's environment. Despite the lessons learned about the weakness of past practices, there is still a conditioned impression in the minds of some of the wider community that requesting a service is associated with substitute care. Many people therefore feel reluctant to seek help at an early stage.

2. The growing numbers of elderly confused people far outweigh the resources that are available. Inevitably service provision priority is directed more towards those in crisis rather than towards those in need - which could perhaps prevent a crisis occurring. Given the relatively low funding priority for psychogeriatric services, the picture is unlikely to change radically in the foreseeable future.

The growing demands for care services, coupled with the reality that traditional residential provision will not suffice, has forced service providers to rethink the types of service that have traditionally been made available.

The closure of long stay wards in psychiatric hospitals, fewer residential homes in the statutory sector and the current financial problems that the residential private care sector is being exposed to, firmly shifts the emphasis of care back into the community. Community-based health care programmes are emerging. They have already become an established and integral part of the service provision available in some areas.

At present there are four main sectors that contribute different kinds of specialised facilities and a diverse range of resources for those diagnosed with dementia. These include:-

The Health Authority	The Voluntary Sector
The Social Services Department	The Private Sector

In the past, each organisation has tended to work in comparative isolation from the others. A client is assessed in relation to the resources and expertise available to that agency and, where appropriate, they have been offered a service or, alternatively, they are passed on to another organisation. Sadly, people with dementia have often been the victims of such an insular approach.

The disease is one that has both medical and psycho-social characteristics. Overworked GPs have often responded to requests for help with responses that direct individuals away from health care resources. *"Social Services can help you, not me"*: this has often been echoed by Health Service workers. The opposite has often been true when people approach Social Services departments. Fortunately, it is becoming more widely recognised that many individuals in need have been shunted to and fro between overworked agencies and, as a result, have often been denied a comprehensive quality service.

Three important objectives have been the focus of much debate in recent years. The first concerns quality assurance. The second is about making services more cost-effective. The third is concerned with a more co-ordinated approach for those with dementia. One response, in an effort to realise these objectives, has been an increase in the co-ordination of services at a funding level. The 'joint funding' of some Health and Social Care services is now well established. These initiatives have played an important part in providing a more comprehensive and multi-disciplinary service. However, despite these efforts, there is a growing recognition that inter-service co-ordination at the fieldwork level needs to be greatly improved in order to ensure that individuals with dementia have a range of services that are co-ordinated in a systematic and consistent way.

There seems little point in preventing the secondary problems associated with moving people away from their homes, if the innovative services that are brought into people's homes also create secondary confusion and disorientation due to lack of proper co-ordination.

Developments: Health Services

Traditionally, the General Practitioner has been seen as the primary co-ordinator of physical care for those with dementia. In recent years, developments in the field of psychogeriatric medicine have significantly changed the way in which elderly people with dementia have been dealt with. Domiciliary visits from specialist doctors to assess and advise General Practitioners about medication, care and management have prevented a number of elderly people being inappropriately medicated and/or admitted to hospital prematurely.

The emergence, in the late sixties and early seventies, of specialist doctors in the field of psychogeriatric medicine gave a new and significant status to the way that elderly people with dementia were approached. This establishment of a specialist service began to challenge traditional views and care practices. Although still not recognised widely enough, the provision of a specialist medical service affirmed that individuals with dementia have a complex range of problems that require specialist knowledge and skills. Sadly, adequate levels of resource provision in respect of this are still found wanting. Many individuals with incurable conditions like dementia are still labelled and managed without having the benefit of a skilled assessment to determine a correct diagnosis. Nonetheless, the presence of a psychogeriatric service has become an integral part of Health Service provision in most areas. Such a presence has brought an improvement on the more primitive methods of care for those with dementia.

Parallel developments in the care of those with dementia are also being more fully realised by other Health Care workers. Some Community Psychiatric Nurses now have specific specialist responsibilities for those elderly individuals referred to the psychogeriatric services. Their primary role and function is to monitor mental health treatment and to administer medication. They are often in a primary position to observe changes and early deterioration. They can often alert and mobilise the appropriate services to prevent acute crises. Many are well trained in listening skills and family counselling. They can be invaluable to carers and individuals with dementia, for emotional support, advice and information about a range of services.

Community Occupational Therapists, can either be employed by the Health Authority or the Social Services Department; some are now employed as specialists in psychiatric occupational therapy. They have an increasing role to play amongst those diagnosed with dementia. Besides assessing people for aids and adaptions to maximise physical functioning, they can be invaluable advisers about reality orientation techniques, reminiscence therapy, and stimulation activities to aid memory retention and minimise disorientation, etc. Occupational therapists, particularly those specialised in working with elderly people, usually have the most up-to-date information on modern aids for people with dementia. Similarly, there is an increasing number of Community Physiotherapists. More and more their work in enabling people to maximise physical functioning is bringing them into contact with elderly people who are confused and/or diagnosed with dementia. Imaginative use of traditional techniques and the developing of new exercises and activities can be of tremendous benefit for those with dementia. Both disciplines recognise the close inter-relatedness of the body and mind as being inseparable to the success of any treatment programme.

Clinical Psychologists have a more recent history in Health Care Services. In some areas, services are available to measure memory retention, etc. Many have contributed to behavioural programmes aimed at modifying difficult and problematic behaviour.

Parallel to this growing recognition of the importance of a multi-disciplinary approach, other developments within the Health Service authenticate a growing sensitivity towards those with mental health problems.

Firstly, the relocation of workers. There is a growing trend towards community-based locations for mental health workers. People can more easily access the service. Secondly is the recognition of the importance of terminology and the effect this can have on workers, carers and those labelled with a disease. Hence the movement towards multi-disciplinary approaches of care, in conjunction with the change of label from 'Psychiatric' to 'Mental Health Services', reflects a move away from a medical model of care towards a more holistic approach. This emphasises a closer inter-relatedness between the social, emotional, cognitive and physical dimensions of a person. -

Despite a real shortage of resource provision, the quality of service provided by the Health Authority for those with dementia is improving.

Developments in Social Services: The Social Worker's View

Ten years ago the response by a Social Services Department to a request for 'help' or 'intervention' with an elderly confused person was simplistic and narrow. If the person was severely confused, wandering, considered a nuisance or at risk in the community, then residential care was seen to be the only response - indeed it was the only real resource available.

Home Helps were working in the more traditional roles of housework, shopping, etc. Work was task-orientated, with Home Helps often only being allocated a few hours a week to a client. Those with dementia who required a daily service could not easily be assisted by remaining in the community. Active and enabling roles with elderly clients, awareness of dementia as a disease and the significance of altered behaviour and ability to care for oneself were scarcely recognised or understood. Thus there was little encouragement for Home Help Organisers to seek education and training to develop an entirely different method of working.

The past few years has witnessed a significant change in Local Authority service provision for elderly people and their relatives. The quality of service provision throughout the country, however, is inconsistent; funding priority for the elderly population varies significantly from area to area.

The education and training of some Social Workers in their knowledge of dementia has improved the quality of initial assessments. Some Local Authority Social Services Departments now have specialist teams specifically to respond to elderly people. Workers can establish a comprehensive knowledge about networks of support services and they can often work closely with other professionals in the same specialised field. However, other Social Services Departments operate a 'patch work' system. Assessments are often carried out by generic workers whose expertise with elderly confused people largely hinges on whether the worker is interested enough or sufficiently motivated to participate in specialised training about elderly people with dementia.

The reorganisation in many areas of Home Help Organisers and Social Workers into single teams, incorporating Occupational Therapists and other specialist workers, has led to more joint assessments. There is a growing recognition that multi-disciplinary and inter-agency co-operation can produce a more creative, skilled and cost-effective approach to providing care packages aimed at meeting people's needs.

Planned residential care for regular short term periods, day care, Home Helps being trained to recognise the importance of enabling people to retain social skills rather than perpetuating the 'doing for' syndrome, are becoming more integral components of the service offered to those who are demented. To reinforce the enabling functions of the traditional Home Help, some Departments have renamed them 'Home Carers'. The concept of the support service has radically changed. If appropriate, Home Carers may visit the client two or three times a day. Where the demands are considerable, examples of team Home Care work are emerging, including health care support and input from voluntary agencies, enabling some very dependent people to remain at home with a seven days-a-week service, often being visited several times a day.

For people living in areas where such initiatives are already established, services offered today would be markedly different to those offered to people in areas where more traditional service approaches still prevail.

The Voluntary Sector

Historically the voluntary sector has, in the main, provided residential care for those elderly people who need assistance with physical disabilities. Like the Local Authority, they are now faced with the problem that many of their residents are living longer and the problems associated with residents developing dementia can be pronounced.

The debate about whether people with dementia should be segregated or integrated with elderly people who are mentally alert is ongoing. The thorny question surrounds whose rights and choices are to be respected. Should priority be given to:

- the rights of residents who do not want their day-to-day lives affected by some of the behaviours that may manifest themselves with the onset of dementia in their fellow-residents, or
- the rights of the individual with dementia who may want to remain in their familiar residential environment?

Besides being providers of residential care, voluntary agencies have a well-established reputation for providing support services, particularly for carers. Support groups for those who care for a relative with dementia are growing all over the country. The voluntary sector's provision of practical home support services is among the most imaginative to be found anywhere - largely because the role and function of voluntary agencies is not defined by statute, allowing them to provide complementary services to fill the gaps in the statutory provision of services by Health Authorities and Social Services Departments.

The Private Sector

Residential provision in the private sector has grown significantly during recent years. Some establishments are specifically for elderly people with dementia, while others are exposed to the problems mentioned above when those with exclusively physical disabilities are integrated with individuals who may exhibit more problem behaviours. The growth in private residential care has directly resulted from funding that has been available from the Department of Social Security and, in some cases, 'top up' funding from the Local Authority. It is difficult to speculate about future developments in the private sector.

The proposed Community Care Act is partially concerned with restructuring the way funding is provided for the private sector. Until the implications of this have been established in terms of financial gain or loss, the rapid increases we have seen in this sector are likely to slow down, at least in the short term. The current uncertainty leaves many existing owners of private residential care very unsure about their future market potential as providers of residential services.

* * * * *

The details listed above are by no means exhaustive in respect of the range of service provision that is available. It is evident that a number of significant developments have taken place during recent years and that the range and the co-ordination of services have markedly improved. For those with dementia, this improvement can have a real impact on the individual's day-to-day experiences. Such developments can also provide a real alternative to residential care. Despite these radical and recent developments, there continues to be significant problems regarding geographical location. Sadly, 'choice' hinges largely on where a person resides and whether the needs of elderly people with dementia have been given any significant funding status.

Chapter Six

Your Questions Answered.

In this final chapter, the more common questions about dementia are posed. They are by no means exhaustive, but they do attempt to bring into sharper focus those issues that are constantly raised by carers and workers.

Is it only elderly people who get dementia?

No. Dementia can have an early onset. Although not common, some people do present with both Alzheimer's disease and multi-infarct dementia as early as 40 to 50 years.

The AIDS virus can also attack the brain. Younger people with the AIDS virus can present with the signs and symptoms of dementia. In the absence of finding a 'cure' for the AIDS virus, the problem is likely to increase.

Also, some fairly rare conditions may cause dementia in younger people, Pick's disease being one. The disease tends to filtrate into the area of the brain that affects judgement. This often manifests itself in impairment of social behaviour.

Are there any known causes for Alzheimer's disease?

During the last 10-15 years, research has been carried out in relation to Alzheimer's disease and current research developments are emerging more rapidly. Of those hypotheses that have been documented, no cause has yet been determined.

Post mortems of sufferers of Alzheimer's disease have revealed that they do have increased amounts of aluminium in their brain. However, this has been ruled out as a singular cause of the disease.

Recent evidence indicates that an enzyme called acetylcholine is deficient in those with Alzheimer's disease. When acetylcholine, found in nerve cells, is released, it acts as a neuro-transmitter to other nerve cells. Those nerve cells associated with memory rely on acetylcholine. Some work has been done to find a substitute substance to replace the deficient enzyme. Progress has not been sufficient to use substitute substances as part of a routine treatment programme for those with Alzheimer's disease. Nonetheless, work is being continued to find a substitute substance which may help to improve the condition, even if measures are not 'curative'.

Some work has been done on the relationship between the immune system and dementia. Does the body's own defence system of those with Alzheimer's disease attack part of the brain rather than acting entirely as a defence system against external agents? There is no reliable evidence from this work which might determine whether or not a faulty immune system is a cause of the disease.

Research on some neurological diseases is focusing on viral hypotheses. Are the causes of some neurological disorders associated with viruses that may lie dormant for years, but then suddenly become active?

At present, little can be done to prevent the onset of the disease; no singular or multi-factorial aetiology has been adequately determined.

What about multi-infarct dementia?

For those with a multi-infarct dementia, more can be done to prevent the problem because the cause is associated with blood supply to the brain. Preventive strategies are concerned with measures taken to reduce the possibility of, for example, strokes, heart attacks, high blood pressure and arterial conditions. Although the dementia cannot be treated once it has manifest itself, there are strategies which can minimise further brain tissue damage and hence mental deterioration.

Is dementia hereditary?

There is no research available to suggest that there is a genetic connection. There is, however, some research indicating that there may be a greater risk of other family members being affected if the onset of the disease started at an early age. For those families who have elderly relatives with the disease, the risk of inheriting dementia is no greater than for relatives who have not been affected by the disease.

Is is possible to catch the disease while looking after somebody who has been diagnosed with dementia?

Dementia, in itself, is not regarded as an infectious disease. It cannot be transmitted from one person to another.

Is there any point in treating other mental health conditions in a person who has been diagnosed with dementia?

Some individuals diagnosed with dementia may have a history of other mental health disorders, e.g. depression, schizophrenia, anxiety state, etc. Characteristic symptoms of these other disorders may well re-emerge, and often do, parallel to the dementia taking its course. These other conditions are treatable and should continue to be treated, where appropriate, despite the presence of dementia. The individual's quality of life can be severely and prematurely impaired if careful assessments are not made as to which symptoms characterise the dementia and which are recurrences of previous mental health problems.

In one psychiatric unit in which I have worked, individuals with dementia were often treated for their re-occurring depressive symptoms because both conditions could prevent functioning at home. Treating their depression enabled many of them to return home and to remain there longer with help, despite the dementia slowly progressing.

Are some groups of people more prone to the disease than others?

Apart from the elderly population, there is no evidence that any one group of the population is more likely to get the disease than any other. Nor is it a disease that is related to geographical location and/or occupation, or any other such factor.

It is often recorded the men are more prone to a multi-infarct dementia. However, there is no evidence, to my knowledge, that suggests that those with a history of other mental disorders are more likely to become afflicted with dementia. As previously mentioned in Chapter One however, there are many incidences where other mental disorders that are treatable are mistaken for dementia.

There are indications that individuals with Downs' syndrome have a higher risk of developing Alzheimer's disease at a relatively young age. Research is continuing in this area of study.

Can people with dementia have one or more forms of the disease?

Yes. Of those people diagnosed with the disease, at least one-fifth of them have both Alzheimer's disease and multi-infarct dementia.

Do people with dementia understand what they are doing?

There appears to be no clear cut answer to this. Some elderly people slip from being autonomous individuals into being totally dependent on others; throughout they appear happy and placid adapting without any signs of distress about behaviour that may appear odd or out of character; for others, however, the distress is very real.

During the early stages of the disease, individuals often know they may have done something out of character but, when asked, they deny it. This is particularly so if they feel that their future autonomy is under threat if they admit to behaving in a strange way. The term that is often used for this is 'confabulation'. Such a strategy is often pronounced in assessment interviews with individuals. Having to cover up for one's own behaviour and the fears that may go with dishonesty can be extremely distressing for the individual during the early stages of the disease. If one's concept of one's behaviour is linked with being segregated and removed from home, it is hardly surprising that there may be an attempt to conceal problems.

As the disease progresses, individuals may have less cognitive understanding that at times they have behaved in a way that is out of character. Their emotional responses indicate that they may be painfully aware that something is happening to them that appears outside their ability to control. They may, for example be very tearful, angry or frustrated. As detailed in Chapter Two, distress may be revealed through behaviour rather than expressed through speech.

Can tests be carried out to confirm the presence of dementia?

At present no medical tests are available to confirm an individual has Alzheimer's disease, except via a post mortem. However, a number of tests can be carried out to eliminate other conditions, the symptoms of which could mimic Alzheimer's disease.

A diagnosis of Alzheimer's disease is generally based on information given about the person, their previous patterns of living and current changes that are observed at the time of assessment. In some cases, a series of questions are used to measure, for example, memory retention, powers of concentration, etc.

Those who are in close proximity to elderly people have an important contribution to make in the assessment processes. The rate of onset, in what part of the day the person is confused, what the person becomes disorientated about, small changes in behaviour, eating and sleep patterns, etc. can be very meaningful in determining a diagnosis.

Can a person who has dementia hand over the management of their financial affairs to a relative or friend.

It depends to a large extent on the individual's mental capabilities. If the individual concerned is capable of fully understanding the powers they are handing over to another person, then a legal document can be drawn up.

Power of Attorney gives responsibility to a designated person to act on behalf of somebody who is not in a position to manage their financial affairs. The appointed person is usually a relative, solicitor, close friend or a bank manager. The designated person has a responsibility to act in the person's best interests. Their actions must be "in respect of" and not "in spite of" the person who has designated their authority.

'Designated authority' can range from giving a person authority for a specific purpose over a limited period of time, to giving authority to somebody to manage all their affairs for an indefinite period of time. It is important to ensure that any agreement reached is recorded on the appropriate forms, which can be obtained from a solicitor. Power of Attorney is open to a great deal of abuse, particularly if broad and indefinite powers are designated. People with dementia can be extremely vulnerable.

Power of Attorney cannot be used and should not be used if the individual does not fully understand what they are doing. In law, they would not be deemed mentally competent; the document would be deemed invalid. Solicitors involved in drawing up documents may well require medical confirmation about the individual's level of competence, particularly if there is any doubt about the person's mental capabilities.

In the past, a Power of Attorney made while a person was able to understand would be regarded as invalid once a person reaches a stage where they would not understand the original agreement made. In 1985, the law changed on this matter. If a designated person is appointed during a time when the individual concerned was able to understand, the Power of Attorney continues to operate.

If a person owns a house or has capital assets, such as savings, and they are not competent either to manage their affairs or to transfer authority in the way described above, then the Court of Protection should be approached.

The Court of Protection is an office of the Supreme Court. It has a responsibility to protect and manage property where mental disorder prevents an individual from doing so. The powers of the Court of Protection are detailed in Part VII of the Mental Health Act 1983.

The Court of Protection can appoint what is known as a Receiver; this could be, for example, a family member, a solicitor, the Local Authority or an official of the Court of Protection. The Receiver is given the authority to manage the person's affairs under the supervision of the Court of Protection, thus offering dementia sufferers maximum protection of their affairs.

An application has to be supported with a medical certificate confirming that the individual concerned is incapable of managing their own affairs by reason of a mental disorder described in the Mental Health Act 1983. The application can be made by a relative with the help of a solicitor through the Personal Applications section of the Court. The Court also requires from the applicant details about the client's assets and outstanding debts.

The client is served with a notice about the proceedings and has seven days to object. She/he can also express an opinion as to the way their affairs should be dealt with. The client or any person affected by the Court's decision has the right of appeal.

An administration fee is payable to the Court of Protection. Despite the cost and the time it may take to process this kind of application, it is an important and necessary step, particularly where there is real concern about an individual's assets being misappropriated.

Can a person with dementia be removed from their home against their will?

Yes, in certain circumstances. If the person concerned is considered to be suffering from a mental disorder defined in the Mental Health Act 1983 and they need hospital admission for his/her own health and safety or for the safety of others, then an application can be made to have the individual admitted to hospital for a specified period of time. Procedures for this kind of intervention are detailed in the Mental Health Act 1983. In the main, this is not a course of action that would be generally used for people with dementia. The risks to either the individual concerned or others would have to be extreme.

Although not commonly used, a Guardianship Order can also be applied for under the aegis of the Mental Health Act 1983. Among its powers, a Guardianship Order gives the appointed Guardian the power to require an individual to reside in a specified place. The Guardian appointed may be a relative, the Local Authority Social Services Department or somebody who is regarded suitable to execute the powers and functions of a Guardian. Section 7 of the Mental Health Act 1983 details the procedures in relation to Guardianship Orders.

Bibliography

Ackerman, N. J. (1966) "Treating the Troubled Family", Basic Books, New York

Argyle, M. (1987) "The Psychology of Happiness", Methuen, London

Beech, D. (1986) "Social Work and Mental Disorder", PEPAR Publications

Brearly, G. and Birchley, P. (1986) "Introducing Counselling Skills and Techniques", Faber and Faber, London

Carver, V. and Liddiard, P. (editors), (1978) "An Aging Population", Open University Press

Hicks, C. (1988) "Who Cares", Virago Press

Kubler-Ross, E. (1970) "On Death and Dying", Tavistock, London

Lascelles, R. V. (1985) "Coping with Loss", PEPAR Publications

Marris, P. (1974) "Loss and Change", Routledge & Kegan Paul Ltd.

Munro, A. and McCulloch, W. (1969) "Psychiatry for Social Workers", Pergamon Press

Parkes, C. M. (1972) "Studies of Grief in Adult Life", International Universities Press, New York

Rimmer, L. (1982) "Reality Orientation Principles and Practice", Winslow Press

Strutton, S. (1989) "Counselling Older People", Hodder & Stoughton

Walrond-Skinner, S. (1988) "Family Matters", SPCK

Wattis, Dr J. P. (1988) "Confusion in Old Age", Equation in association with the British Medical Association

Worden, W. J. (1983) "Grief Counselling & Grief Therapy", Tavistock Publications Ltd

Wright, F. (1986) "Left to Care Alone", Gower, London

Appendix One

Useful Organisations

Listed below are names, addresses and telephone numbers of some organisations that may be helpful for carers and workers. Some of them have groups in many different geographical locations throughout the country. Information about these can usually be obtained through the national organisations listed below, local libraries and / or local Citizens' Advice Bureaux.

Alzheimer's Disease Society, 158 Balham High Road, London SW12 9BN, Telephone 081 675 6557

Age Concern England, Astral House, 1268 London Road, London, SW16 4ER, Telephone 081 679 8000

Age Concern Scotland, 33 Castle Street, Edinburgh EH2 3DN, Telephone 031 225 5000

Age Concern Wales, 4th Floor, 1 Cathedral Road, Cardiff CF1 9SD, Telephone 0222 371 821

Age Concern Northern Ireland, 6 Lower Crescent, Belfast BT7 1NR, Telephone 0232 245729

Association of Continence Advisers, Disabled Living Foundation, 380-384 Harrow Road, London W9 2HU, Telephone 071 289 6111

Association of Crossroads Attendant Schemes Ltd, 10 Regent Place, Rugby, Warwickshire CV21 2PN, Telephone 0788 573 653

Carers National Association, 29 Chilsworth Mews, London W2 3RG, Telphone 071 724 7776

Centre on Environment for the Handicapped, 35 Great Smith Street, London SW1P 3BJ, Telephone 071 222 7980

Chest, Heart and Stroke Association, CHSA House, 123-127, Whitecross Street, London EC1Y 8JJ, Telephone 071 490 7999

Court of Protection, Stewart House, 24 Kingsway, London WC2B 6JX, Telephone 071 269 7358

Cruise Bereavement Care, Cruise House, 126 Sheen Road, Richmond, Surrey TW9 1UR, Telephone 081 940 4818

Centre for Policy on Ageing, 25-31 Ironmonger Row, London EC1V 3QP, Telephone 071 253 1787

Dial UK (Disablement Information and Advice Lines), Victoria Buildings, 117 High Street, Clay Cross, Chesterfield, Derbyshire S45 9DZ, Telephone 0246 250055

Disabled Living Foundation, 380-384 Harrow Road, London W9 2HU, Telephone 071 289 6111

Department of Social Security - freeline, a confidential advice on all benefits, Telephone 0800 666 555

Help the Aged, 16/18 St James' Walk, London EC1R 0BE, Telephone 071 253 0253

Holiday Care Service, 2 Old Bank Chambers, Station Road, Horley, Surrey RH6 9HW, Telephone 0293 774535

Mental Health Foundation, 8 Hallam Street, London W1N 6DH, Telephone 071 580 0145

Mind (National Association of Mental Health), 22 Hartley Street, London W1N 2ED, Telephone 071 637 0741

Appendix Two

Useful Books about Practical Aspects of Care

Alzheimer's Disease Society (1984) "Caring for the Person with Dementia"; a guide for families and other carers (see useful organisations for address)

Holden, U. (1984) "Reality Orientation Reminders"; pocket reference of ideas, Winslow Press, Telford Road, Bicester, Oxon OX6 0TS, Telephone 0869 244 733

Holden, U., Martin, C. and White, M. (1984) "Twenty Four Hour Approach to the Problems of Confusion in Elderly People", Winslow Press (see address above)

Kohner, N. (1988) "Caring at Home" - a handbook for people looking after someone at home, Kings Fund Centre, 126 Albert Street, London NW1 7NF

Lodge, B. (1981) "Coping with Caring", Mind (see Appendix 1 for address)

Mace, N. L. and Rabins, P. (1985) "The 36 Hour Day", Age Concern and Hodder & Stoughton (available from bookshops)

Murphy, E. (1986) "Dementia and Mental Illness in the Old"; a practical guide, Macmillan Papermac Health (available from bookshops)

Rimmer, L. (1982) "Reality Orientation - Principles and Practice", Winslow Press (see address above)

Stokes, G. (1986) "Aggression - Common Problems with the Elderly Confused", Winslow Press (see address above)

Stokes, G. (1987) "Incontinence & Inappropriate Urinating", Winslow Press (see address above)

Stokes, G. (1986) "Screaming and Shouting", Winslow Press (see address above)

Stokes, G. (1986) "Wandering", Winslow Press (see address above)

Appendix Three

Useful Publications about Finance

"Claiming a Supplementary Pension Towards the Fees of a Registered Private or Voluntary Home", (1987), Counsel and Care for the Elderly, Lower Ground Floor, Twyman House, 16 Bonny Street, London NW1 9PG

"Disability Rights Handbook (1989/90)", Disability Alliance, 25 Denmark Street, London WC2H 8NJ, Telephone 071 240 0806

"Enduring Powers of Attorney", Court of Protection (see Appendix 1 for address)

Gostin, L. (1983) "Court of Protection", Mind Publications (see Appendix 1 for address)

"Legal Aid Guide", Legal Aid Head Office, Newspaper House, 8-16 Great New Street, London EC4 3BN

"Making the Most of the Court of Protection", (1987), Kings Fund Centre, 126 Albert Street, London NW1 7NF, Telephone 071 267 6111

Mind (1988), "A-Z of Welfare Benefits for People with Mental Illness", Mind Publications Department (see Appendix 1 for address)

"Your Rights", (published yearly) Age Concern (see Appendix 1 for address)

Index

Acetycholine, 51
Age Concern, 59
Aggression, 20
AIDS, 51
Alcohol intoxification, 9
Alzheimer's Disease, 14, 51, 59
Anger, carer's, 29
Anxiety, 11
Assessment:-
   Compulsory, 57
   Families, 32-34
Association of Continence
   Advisers, 59
Association of Crossroads
   Attendants, 59
Assumptions, 7, 15, 24, 34, 42

Behaviour, attention-seeking,
   16-22
Behaviour, a framework for
   understanding, 24
Bereavement, 10-11

Carers, National Association, 59
Centre for Policy on Ageing, 60
Centre on Environment for the
   Handicapped, 59
Chest, Heart and Stroke
   Association, 59
Communications with the
   confused, 39-40
Community psychiatric nurse,
   46
Confusion, causes, 7-15

Constipation, 23
Court of Protection, 55
Cruise, 60

Delusions, 23
Dementia, 14-15, 52-55
Department of Social Security,
   60
Depression, 11-12
Diagnosis - impact on others, 28
DIAL UK, 60
Disabled Living Foundation, 60
Downs' Syndrome &
   Alzheimer's Disease, 53

Emotional factors, 17-18
Emotional needs, 17
Environmental Stimuli, 36-38
Exercise, 16-17

Family Systems:
   Boundaries, 33
   Decision-making, 33
   Links with the environment,
   33-34
   Problem-solving, 33
Financial Affairs of the confused,
   55

General Practitioners, 45
Group activities, 41
Guardianship Orders, 57
Guilt, carer's, 30

Hallucinations, 23
Health Authority Services, 45
Helplessness, 31
Help the Aged, 60
Holiday Care Service, 60

Immune System, 52
Incontinence, 19-20
Interpersonal stimuli, 38-41

Loss of inhibition, 16-17

Medication, side effects, 9
Memory loss, 8-14
   helping, 36-42
Mental Health Act 1983, 56
Mental Health Foundation, 60
Mental influences, disorders, 12-13, 23, 52, 53
Mind, 60
Multi-infarct dementia, 15

Occupational Therapist, 46-47, 48

Paraphrenia, 13
Physical influences on
   confusion, 8-9
Physical influences, 17
Physiotherapist, 47
Pick's disease, 51
Power of Attorney, 56
Private sector provision, 50

Psychiatric assessments, 12
Psychogeriatric services, 46

Reality Orientation, 35
   Individual/group, 35-36
Responses to confusion:
   Families, 27
   Neighbours, 25-26
Risk-taking, 18

Social Services provision, 48-49

Treatment of confusion, 8, 11, 13, 14

Voluntary sector provision, 49-50

Wandering, 16-17